Stop Making

THESE FASHION MISTAKES

Stop Making
THESE FASHION MISTAKES

A quick style guide that can instantly break
the cycle of feeling like you look 'okay' and
'good enough' to looking proportionate,
empowered and self-confident.

by
HOLLY KATZ

INTRODUCTION

Is your image holding you back?

By reading this captivating and quick style guide, you can instantly break the cycle of feeling like you look "okay" and "good enough" to feeling proportionate, empowered, and self-confident.

This book describes in detail the top fashion and style mistakes that people make without even knowing it. While learning these short style principles, you will soon understand why keeping your closet out of chaos, wearing the correct fitting undergarments, and dressing according to your lifestyle, age, and body type will evolve your personal style.

Getting dressed is something that should add joy and confidence to your everyday life. Through fashion and style, you have complete control over the message you are sending to the world.

Use these tactics to instantly change how you feel about your image without losing weight or spending money on new clothes. While not every day is a home run, you do have the option to "opt-in" and dress the way that makes you feel like authentically you. This book is the first step in your style evolution to becoming "unstuck." Congratulations on making your outside match your inside. I mean, I don't know how your day can get any better?

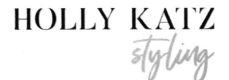

Stop Making
THESE FASHION MISTAKES

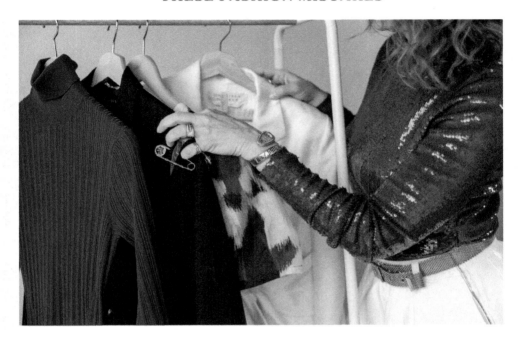

TABLE OF CONTENTS

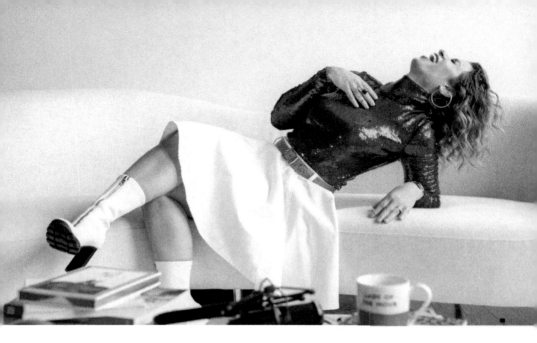

MEET HOLLY KATZ

The best friend you never knew you needed in fashion, Holly Katz is an Atlanta and Manhattan–based personal stylist, fashion writer, and host of the popular Fashion Crimes Podcast.

She's featured often in national media including the Associated Press, InStyle, Marie Claire, Glam.com, The Knot, Newsday, The Washington Post, and Yahoo.com.

Holly boasts an impressive client list including celebrities, television networks, ad agencies, photographers, and publishers. She is frequently invited to speak by companies looking to polish their employees' professional image.

Holly transforms the lives of her clients and empowers them by leading them through her step–by–step personal styling process. Holly is the ultimate style coach, whose clients always say they wish they had hired her years earlier.

Learn more at:

www.hollykatzstyling.com
www.fashioncrimespodcast.com

The 1st Most Common Fashion Mistake

DRESSING TOO YOUNG OR TOO OLD FOR YOUR AGE

Most people dress according to their mood. For example, if you're feeling upbeat and energetic, you might put a little more effort into getting dressed and feeling good about yourself.

If you are feeling down and lacking energy, you might dress for comfort in oversized, loose clothing that may or may not be presentable.

But here's the thing; **society is superficial whether you like it or not, or whether you believe it or not.** It takes three seconds for someone to judge you before you get a chance to say a word.

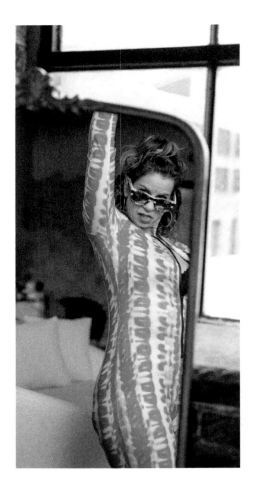

DRESSING TOO YOUNG OR TOO OLD

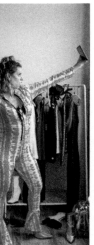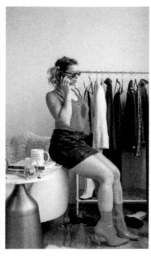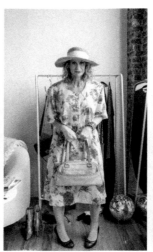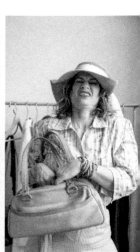

Even though style is subjective, developing and evolving your style takes years. When starting out, you must consider your age, lifestyle, life phase, industry, and area where you live when deciding what to buy.

If these things aren't taken into consideration when shopping, then your style will not reflect the person you are today. And that really is the point, isn't it? To have an image that attracts positive energy and exudes self-confidence for the person you are today?

DRESSING TOO OLD

When you leave your house, your clothes dictate the message that you are sending to others.

If you don't take the opportunity to dress with intention, you can slide into a style comfort zone that is difficult to break out of.

What defines dressing as "too old" for your current age?

- Clothes that are usually sold in big box and department stores that are marketed to the "mature or value customer." You can usually tell by the displays, the models in print or the type of people you see shopping in that section or store.

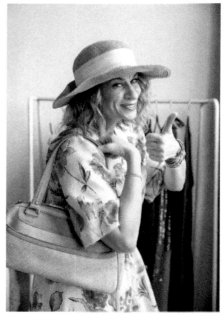

- If comfort and/or functionality are more important than the shape, silhouette, or style of the garment.

- If you dress according to what people 15/20 years older than you are wearing.

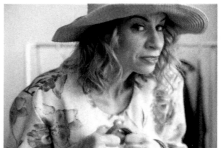

- If you're wearing what your parents/family/spouse tells you to wear, or you let them make style choices for you.

DRESSING TOO YOUNG

When people don't want to grow up, consciously or unconsciously, most likely their wardrobe will reflect this.

It's not uncommon for people to rebel with their clothing choices if they feel they are being forced into adulthood. Transitioning into post-college life can be challenging when you have a lower starting salary and a limited budget.

Spending money on clothes may seem like a last priority. However, when you invest in quality clothing at the beginning of your career, you'll build a wardrobe and evolve your style as you age.

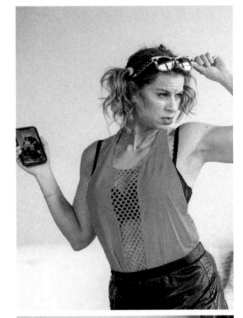

If you don't evolve your style each year, you might become stuck in a style rut, leading you to wear the same clothing from 10 or 15, or 20 years prior.

 HOT TIP

Evolving your style leads you to clean out your closet slowly and on the regular, so you don't end up purging everything you own in one day because you haven't shopped in 15 years.

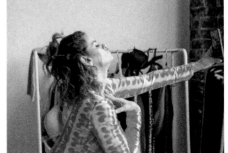

The 2nd Most Common Fashion Mistake

WEARING INCORRECT, NON-EXISTENT, OR ILL-FITTING UNDERGARMENTS

When working with clients, I see this time and time again.

People who opt out, or aren't sure how to wear the right undergarments will have a more difficult time finding clothes that fit properly. In most cases, this leads to guessing and/or wearing the wrong size bra which is the **ultimate** fashion crime.

Wearing the correct size bra is something so simple that can make or break how you feel in your clothes.

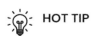 **HOT TIP**

Not giving yourself a chance to wear the right size bra will give you an incorrect or "skewed" image of yourself in the mirror.

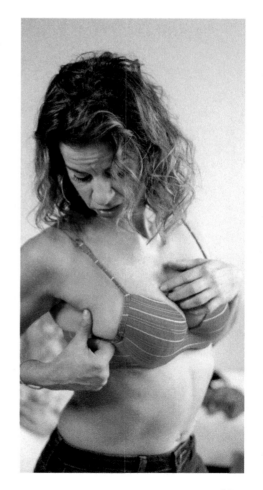

TYPES OF SHAPEWEAR

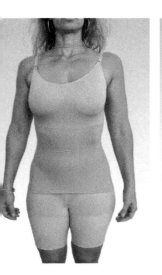 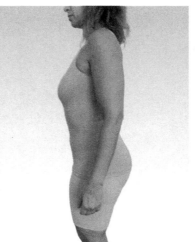 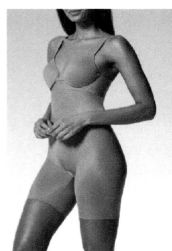

When you have the support you need underneath, you can't help but exude confidence like never before in your clothes. Wearing shapewear is a powerful advantage that puts your curves in all the right places.

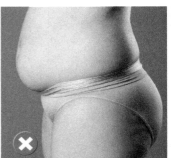

It's a style tool I use to feel my best. This is a product that's considered an important part of a functional wardrobe, especially if someone needs a little extra help underneath.

Also, it's a fantastic way to manipulate stubborn areas without having to constantly feel insecure about your body, or feel that you need to lose weight.

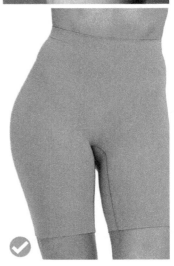

SOLUTION:

ALWAYS GET FITTED FOR A BRA

One of the biggest fashion problems that women face is wearing the incorrect size bra.

This can happen easily during and after pregnancy, significant life cycles, and of course, aging.

The breasts should lie on the inside frame of your body. Not out to the side, spilling over the top of the cups, or lying flat hanging down.

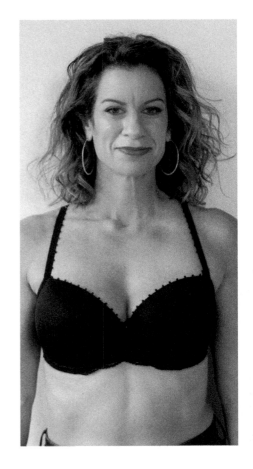

They should be held up and together to give the illusion of a smaller waist.

As a woman's body changes throughout her lifetime, and/or if there is a significant weight change, it's crucial that she gets fitted and re-measured for a bra every year or so. If your weight is consistent, then you should still make sure to get fitted every 2–3 years by a professional.

BRA FITTING

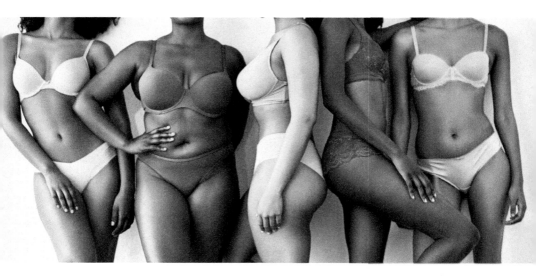

Bras need to be replaced every 12–18 months, depending on how often they are worn and washed. This is due to the wear over time of the elastic in the straps and band. The elastic gets stretched out and is less supportive over time.

To get maximum support, care for your bras by washing them on delicate and then laying them flat to dry. To look the best you possibly can in your clothes, wearing the right size bra is a game-changer!

The 3rd Most Common Fashion Mistake

NOT DRESSING FOR YOUR BODY TYPE

Body image is one of the most common complaints people have that are struggling with style.

Whether people love their body or not, they will find some minute flaw to complain about. If they hate their body image, then most use that as an excuse to stick to their current style.

Understanding and appreciating your body for what it does for you will turn your negative self-talk into positive. Also, wearing clothes that fit your body properly will offer the support you need to look your best in your clothes.

 HOT TIP

Wearing clothes that are too big make you look bigger, not smaller. Wearing clothes that are too tight make you appear larger, not smaller.

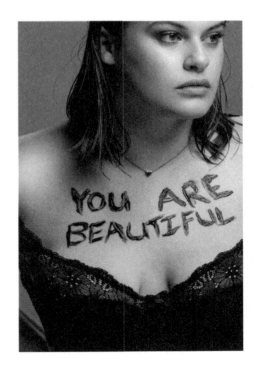

WHAT IS YOUR BODY TYPE?

Your body type is determined by where you carry most of your weight. Measure around your bust, waist and hips, and whichever is the largest measurement determines your body type. If all three measurements are the same or almost the same, then your body type is "straight" or "no curves."

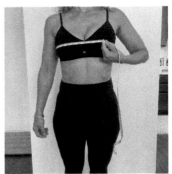

Know this: Clothing that fits your body properly (at any size) can change the reflection in the mirror and the mind.

With structured clothes that hold their shape, it's easy to emphasize what you like about your body.

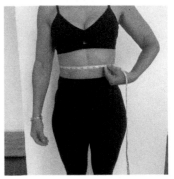

For example, if you think your waist is your best feature, you can wear an A-line skirt or dress with a wider belt to create the illusion of a smaller waist.

If your legs are your best feature, then wearing a dressier short with a heel can show your shapely legs and give you a longer, leaner look.

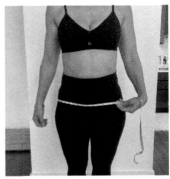

NOT DRESSING FOR YOUR BODY TYPE

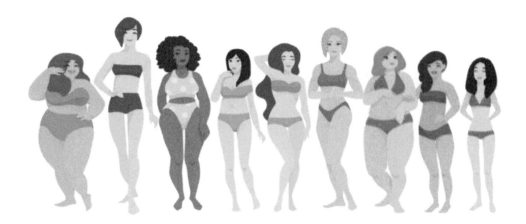

You are not dressing for your body type if:

- You shop for price instead of fit (only shop for things on sale).
- You wear clothes that are too large to hide your body.
- You wear clothes that are too tight or ill-fitting.
- You don't get fitted for a bra or don't wear a bra.
- You wear dated clothing from an era of "who you used to be."
- You wear hand-me-downs/clothing from others, regardless of their style and fit.
- You dress strictly for function and/or comfort.
- You never shop for new clothing, ever.

SOLUTION:

DRESS FOR WHO YOU ARE TODAY

"Dress for the person you are TODAY. Not ten pounds from now, not twenty pounds from yesterday, but the person you are today."

The easiest way to start is to answer what I like to call the "who, what, when, where, why" of you. Answer these questions below:

- Who are you?
- What is your life phase?
- Where are you in your life today?
- What do you need?
- What do you like?
- What do you want?
- Why do you need to make this change?
- Where do you live?
- What industry are you in?

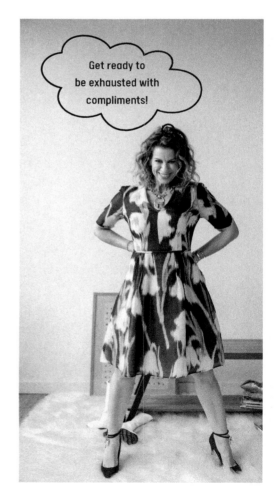

SOLUTION:

DRESS WITH INTENTION

Style is subjective and must make sense for you in your current life phase, industry and lifestyle.

It's a balance between figuring out what you like, what you need, and your budget.

If executed well, style can be used to express yourself in a way that attracts people to you.

It's human nature for others to make a three second quick judgement about you, just by the way you look. By exuding confidence through your style, you'll notice people showing interest and wanting to engage with you. This is one way for you to speak volumes without saying a word.

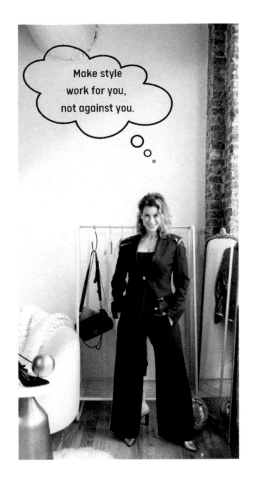

Make style work for you, not against you.

 HOT TIP

When you dress with intention, you look forward to getting dressed, instead of dreading it.

The 4th Most Common Fashion Mistake

DO YOU HAVE CLOSET CHAOS?

Clothes are energy.

They must present themselves to you in a way that makes sense to your eyes and your mind. If they aren't hanging in your closet in a way so that you can quickly recognize what you have, then you aren't going to take the time to figure it out when getting dressed. Things end up just hanging there in limbo...for YEARS, often with the tags still attached, never worn.

This is another serious fashion crime.

Sometimes, people think they have nothing to wear, so new items are purchased.

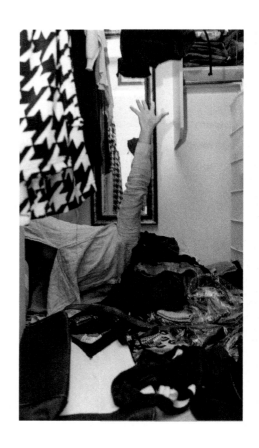

If said items don't get worn right away, they sink into the abyss of the closet chaos only to be found later... usually much, much later.

This is a vicious cycle of compulsive shopping because you have too many items to sift through when trying to get dressed in a timely manner.

COMMON CAUSES OF CLOSET CHAOS

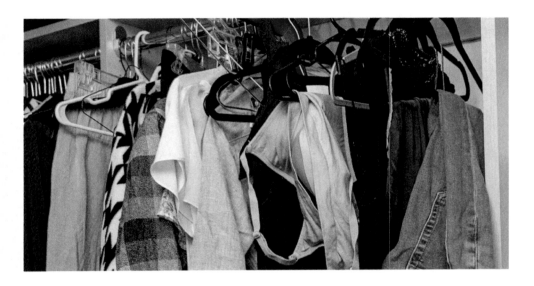

DISORGANIZATION

This might seem obvious, but if you don't have a system of where to find things, it's simply harder to put a cohesive look together.

However, if you think you're organized and you still can't find anything to wear, or it's taking you too long to get dressed, then you probably need some updated organizational practices.

Knowing the best care and storage practices for your clothes will give your items a longer life and keep them looking newer for longer.

SOLUTION:

GAME-CHANGER: CHANGE YOUR HANGERS

JUST SAY NO to plastic, tube, wooden or wire hangers. These take up the maximum amount of space on your hanging bar and will create hanger "bumps" or creases in fabrics.

JUST SAY YES to velvet, slim-line hangers that give you the maximum space for hanging clothes and do not create indentions or creases.

When you change things over to velvet hangers, you will not only save room, but your space will also look so much more organized. Doing just this one thing will change your mindset when getting dressed.

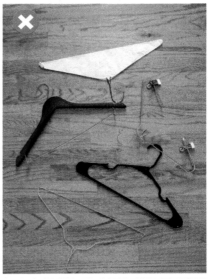

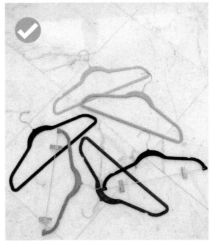

INCONSISTENT LAUNDRY PRACTICES

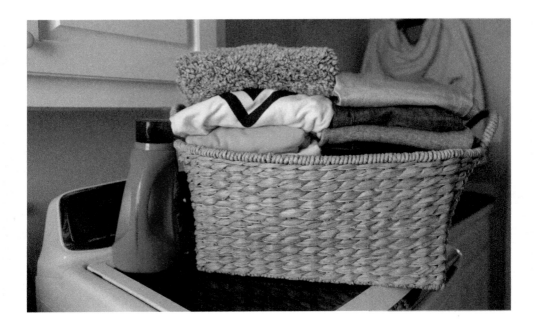

If there isn't a solid plan for who does the laundry in your home, it can lead to closet chaos. Believe it or not, this is one of the most important things that can make or break your style.

After cleaning, your clothes need to come back in a timely manner and present themselves to you. If the laundry isn't done, the dry-cleaning piles up, or if your clean laundry isn't put away, then you'll be constantly looking for your clothes and wasting time.

Having these tasks pile up means there is a disconnect between you and how your clothes can serve you. **In the same way, everything in your kitchen has its place, your closet should be no different.**

It can certainly make or break the start of your day!

SOLUTION

BE CONSISTENT

Schedule time in your calendar to execute the laundry.

Schedule pick-up and delivery of dry-cleaning to get this off your plate.

Planning in this way will hold you accountable to make sure it's done each week.

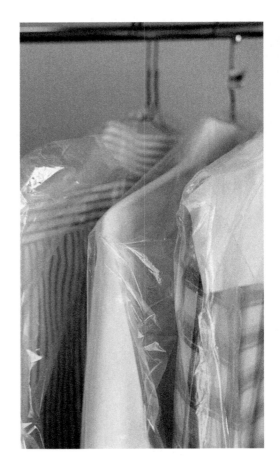

 ## LAUNDRY TIPS

What should be washed? Towels, sheets, workout clothes, pajamas, socks, underwear, t-shirts and jeans.

What should be dry cleaned? Dresses, button down shirts, slacks, jackets, skirts, coats, etc.

Even if you have something that can be washed – like a cotton dress – it could benefit from going to the cleaners so it can be pressed. DO NOT put everything you own in the wash or put everything you own into the dry cleaners. Read care labels to ensure proper care of your clothing.

LIMITED SPACE

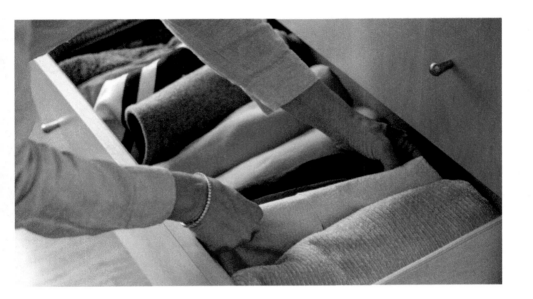

If you share your closet space with a partner, or if your closet is tiny, then knowing what to hang and what to fold is of utmost importance. Having a large dresser or shelving that can hold your folded clothes is a must.

Knowing how to get the most out of your drawer space by folding your items so they stand vertically in the drawers will help.

- Never store excess clothing under your bed or in the garage.
- Do not "seasonally" switch out your clothes. Everything should be readily available to you at all times.
- If you have too many clothes and not enough space, you have too many clothes.
- If you have clothes stored all over the house and in other rooms, you have too many clothes.

SOLUTION:

PROPER STORING TECHNIQUES

Once you change all your hangers to the velvet slimline hangers, you are halfway there.

Fold clothes in a way to guarantee maximum storage space in each drawer. No need to worry, keeping your drawers organized is easy, and you will now be able to see where the garment belongs when it's removed from the drawer.

QUICK TIP 1: Things that should be hung (using velvet slimline hangers): Button downs, slacks, dresses, blouses, skirts, coats, formal wear, etc.

QUICK TIP 2: Things that should be folded: T-shirts, jeans, shorts, sweaters, sweatshirts, workout clothes, socks, underwear, sleepwear, bathing suits, etc.

LUCKY TIP: If you are lucky enough to have extra space, feel free to hang T-shirts and jeans!

Do not store shoes in shoe boxes. They take up valuable storage space and collect dust. It's not considered best closet practices.

SOLUTION:

PROPER FOLDING
TECHNIQUE

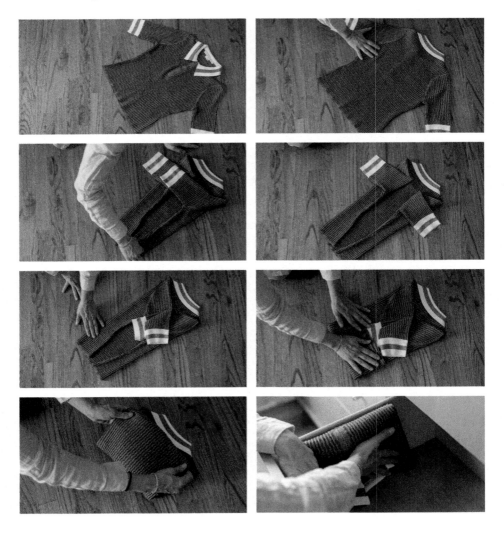

SOLUTION:

NEED EXTRA STORAGE?

You don't have extra room in your closet, but you have extra space?

Purchasing an extra portable closet or extra garment rack can help with the overflow if your wardrobe is larger than your storage space.

DON'T DO THIS: Shoes should be on shoe racks or in over-the-door shoe bags, never in shoes boxes. Nothing should ever be stored under the bed.

And before you fight for your shoe boxes, know this: if your shoes aren't "out" for you to see, the less likely they are to be worn.

Paring your wardrobe down and cleaning out your closet should be completed on the regular if limited space is an issue.

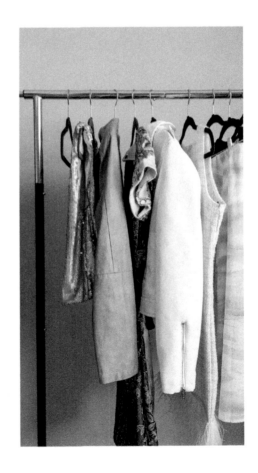

OVER SHOPPING OR COMPULSIVE SHOPPING

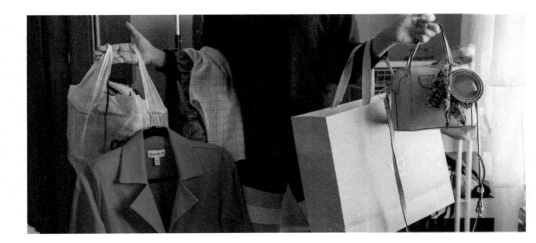

Could you or someone you know be a compulsive shopper? These are the most common traits of a compulsive shopper:

- Buying things you don't need, or way more than you need, because they are "on sale."
- Replacing items on the regular because you can't find them.
- Using shopping as an activity to pass the time.
- Buying things for other people that they don't need to justify the spend.
- Feeling a sense of accomplishment or a "shopper's high" after purchasing.
- Shopping several days per week.
- Living above your means.
- Going into debt because of your shopping habits.
- Cluttering up your space due to the number of items you are bringing home.
- Shopping online in private to avoid judgment.
- Opening several store accounts to spread the debt and/or hide the purchases.

Overshopping or compulsive shopping is the fastest way to closet chaos. If you are bursting out of your closet, you might be over-shopping. Having multiples of items that you don't need or keeping a rainbow of sizes in your closet will also cause extreme organizational issues. Streamlining your clothing only leads to finding your clothes in less time each morning.

SOLUTION:

THE FIRST STEP IS AWARENESS

Realizing you have a habit of compulsive shopping is the first step. Whether you choose to rectify this, is the next step.

A complete closet cleanout to reveal the truth about how much you own, is another way to become aware.

Once you realize how much you have, usually alarm bells go off and the guilt begins. When you keep shopping without taking current inventory, your shopping habit may turn into a bigger issue.

By understanding what you already own, make a style plan for what (and only what) you need. This is just one way to keep you on track from buying excess or extra items you don't need.

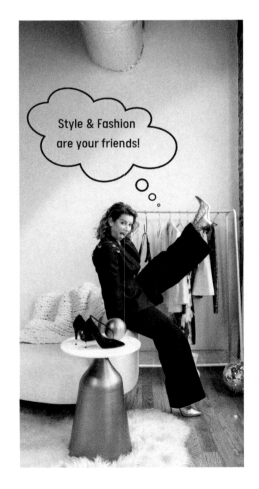

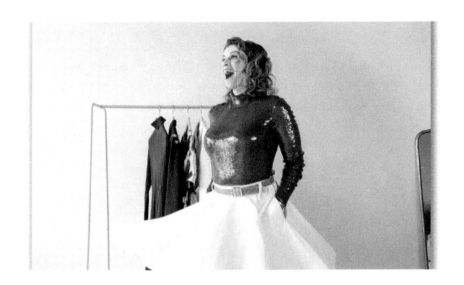

CONGRATULATIONS ON FINISHING YOUR
FIRST FASHION LESSONS!

You are now armed with the most common fashion mistakes to avoid with your own wardrobe.

Regular closet cleanouts and dressing with intention allow you to see what you have and wear the best of the best in your closet.

Properly fitting undergarments are your secret weapon when constructing a cohesive look.

Dressing for the person you are today – with clothes that fit your body type – will raise your vibration and cause you to exude positive energy that is contagious.

People will soon start to notice a little "something different" about you, whether they think you have lost weight or changed your hair. It's really the energy shift that makes style and fashion a tool that you can use to get ahead in life.

(continued...)

Make sure you tune into the Fashion Crimes Podcast every week for more free fashion content. It's all the wardrobe, shopping, and style advice you need to evolve your style with your age. Poof! You look fabulous.

FASHION BESTIES ONLY
EXTRA CONTENT

HOLLY KATZ

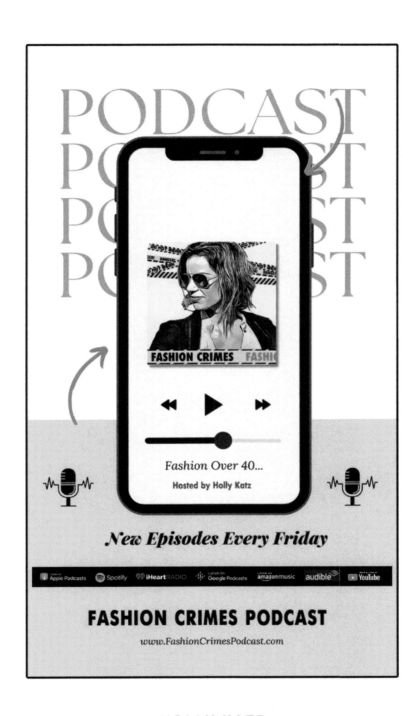

FASHION CRIMES PODCAST

www.FashionCrimesPodcast.com

HOLLY KATZ

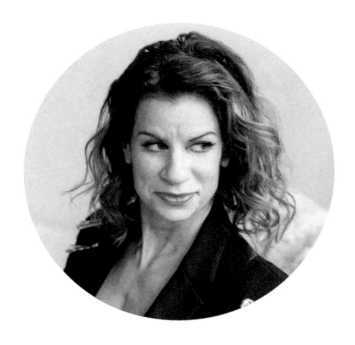

HOLLY KATZ

Personal Styling Services

holly@hollykatzstyling.com

HOLLY KATZ

THE ONLY WARDROBE CHECKLIST YOU WILL EVER NEED

HOLLY KATZ *styling*

UNDERGARMENTS

- [ ] Bras
- [ ] Seamless underwear
- [ ] Shine appliances & sink
- [ ] Shapewear (if needed)

BODYSUITS

- [ ] All Sleeve Lengths
- [ ] Black
- [ ] White
- [ ] Nude

CAMISOLES

- [ ] Black
- [ ] White
- [ ] Nude

T-SHIRTS

- [ ] Novelty / Band / Solid
- [ ] Workout / Exercise

BLOUSES

- [ ] Long Sleeve
- [ ] 3/4 Sleeve
- [ ] Elbow Length
- [ ] Short Sleeve
- [ ] Cap Sleeve
- [ ] Sleeveless

SWEATERS

- [ ] All Sleeve Lengths
- [ ] Pullovers
- [ ] Cardigans
- [ ] Sweatshirts
- [ ] Turtlenecks

JEANS

- [ ] Black
- [ ] Colored
- [ ] Denim (light and dark)

SLACKS

- [ ] Colored
- [ ] Neutral
- [ ] Black

LEGGINGS

- [ ] Faux Leather black
- [ ] Faux leather colored or pattern

SHORTS

- [ ] Denim
- [ ] Black
- [ ] Colored

SKIRTS

- [ ] Maxi
- [ ] Midi
- [ ] Mini

DRESSES

- [ ] Summer
- [ ] Fall
- [ ] Winter
- [ ] Sweater Dresses
- [ ] Work Dresses
- [ ] Dressier, Nighttime, Date Night, etc.
- [ ] Formal, Black Tie

JACKETS

- [ ] Blazers
- [ ] Denim Jacket
- [ ] Lightweight Leather Jacket

OUTERWEAR

- [ ] Puffer Jacket
- [ ] Dress Coat
- [ ] Trench Coat

SHOES

- [ ] Rec Sneakers
- [ ] Workout Sneakers
- [ ] Flats (ballet or loafers)
- [ ] Boots (cowboy, flat, heeled)
- [ ] Sandals (flat, heeled, wedge, stiletto)
- [ ] Pumps: (black, neutral, metallic)

BAGS

- [ ] Work Tote
- [ ] Medium Everyday Bag
- [ ] Clutch for Night Time
- [ ] Wallet on Chain

JEWELRY

- [ ] Costume Mixed with Real
- [ ] Earrings (studs and statement)
- [ ] Bracelets (stacking and chain link)
- [ ] Rings (stacking and real stones)
- [ ] Necklaces (layering and real metal)

ACCESSORIES

- [ ] Belts: Skinny and Wide
- [ ] Scarves

Contact Holly:

holly@hollykatzstyling.com
@hollykatzstyling on IG and FB
www.hollykatzstyling.com

Follow the Podcast!

FASHION CRIMES PODCAST

www.FashionCrimesPodcast.com

Printed in Great Britain
by Amazon

37338253R00046